PATIENT
HANDBOOK
TO MEDICAL CARE

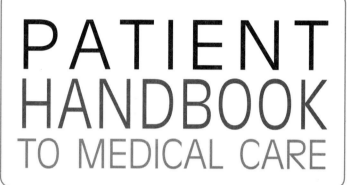

PATIENT HANDBOOK
TO MEDICAL CARE

J. L. Richardson, M.D.

Bend of the River Books
MIAMI, FLORIDA

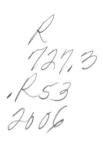

First printing 2006

ISBN-13: 978-0-9771789-2-6
ISBN-10: 0-9771789-2-7
LCCN: 2005931513

ATTENTION CORPORATIONS, UNIVERSITIES, COLLEGES, AND PROFESSIONAL ORGANIZATIONS: Quantity discounts are available on bulk purchases of this book for educational, gift purposes, or as premiums for increasing magazine subscriptions or renewals. Special books or book excerpts can also be created to fit specific needs. For information, please contact Bend of the River Books, P.O. Box 330645, Miami, FL 33233-0645; 866-362-0411.

*Dedicated to
Mom and Dad,
the endless Loves
of my Life.*

TABLE OF CONTENTS

To ensure that you receive the best and even proper medical care, you must know the basics. This book focuses on things that are important when you go to the doctor, and it will help you to obtain the quality medical care you deserve. If you don't know what you're supposed to be getting, you might well not be getting it. I have had many people—family, friends, and patients—tell me that their annual checkup was okay. Then, they describe it. Most of them say their doctor did not ask them the usual questions about their health history and did not do a complete physical examination of their body. They are told that they are okay, yet they commonly receive prescriptions and orders for more tests without knowing why. They may be given an appointment to come back, or they may not.

The goal of this book is to inform and educate patients about medical care. The book is written in an order that corresponds with the basic steps of medical care. The medical records kept by your doctor are the cornerstone of keeping track of everything pertaining to your health. This is one reason why patients should also get copies of their medical records from their doctors. In addition, I suggest that patients keep their own medical records in the form of a diary. Chapter 1 discusses keeping a medical diary and obtaining medical records from your doctors. Chapter 2 outlines what a proper physical exam should include. Preventive medicine guidelines are presented in Chapter 3. Chapter 4 discusses medical tests and what they mean. Chapter 5 describes physician specialists and when they may be necessary. The final chapter discusses types of health insurance and the quality of medical care.

It is very important for patients to learn as much as possible about wellness, disease prevention, and disease management for themselves. In our society we are accustomed to taking a doctor's word on the state of our medical condition and treatment whether or not we understand it and either without asking any questions or without getting adequate answers to the questions we might pose. Today that might not be a healthy situation. It is necessary to be informed to get the most from your health plan and to get the best medical care from the medical resources available in the healthcare system. By reading this book, you will find out how to take charge of your most important asset—you.

This book is written to inform patients about the facts. It is by no means a substitute for your personal physician's care and advice or for that of any of your healthcare providers. Instead, it is a supplement. Use it in good health!

CHAPTER 1

MEDICAL RECORDS AND DIARY

Keeping a medical diary and collecting medical records from each of your doctors will help you stay on top of your medical care and treatment. In today's healthcare system patients tend to see multiple healthcare providers. In addition, contemporary health plans frequently change who these providers are. The medical care system can be frustrating and stressful, no matter which side of it you're on. Keeping track of the vast amount of information that concerns you personally is very important. This book will help you learn what you need to know about going to healthcare providers, which in turn will help you to maintain your own medical diary. Being prepared and informed is the best way you can ensure that you will find and receive the medical care you may need: that is what this patient handbook aims to help you do.

A medical diary is an account of your medical concerns and a record of your doctor visits. In this diary you can record questions and concerns you would like to discuss with your doctor and other healthcare providers. If all of your concerns are not discussed, you will have them on record to discuss at a later time, either in person or by phone, mail, or fax. This will help you keep up with everything, and you will be able to compare your notes with your doctor's. This diary can also be used to record doctor visits, hospital encounters, conversations with your health team, and whatever else you feel is important. With the many doctors one may see over the years, a diary offers a convenient way to keep all the most essential information together. You will find keeping such a diary to be a gratifying experience, as it helps you keep track of your appointments, tests, results, and other things that may be overlooked. Your diary can be handwritten notes in a notebook or it can be typed on a computer or even taped. Blank pages called "My Health Notes" are included at the back of this book to help you get started. The medical diary is a form of healthy self-expression and therapy. Make it a part of your medical plan.

As you begin your medical diary, also take the time to collect your medical records from all the doctors you see. This includes notes from your primary care doctor and specialists, tests, and surgery reports. You may want to start with your primary care doctor, the doctor who sees you the most. To obtain your records, you should submit a medical record release form. This form gives your doctors and other health providers permission to release your records to you. You can also have the records sent directly to your other doctors. This can be done at the doctor's office, by mail, or by fax. You can get a record release form at doctors' offices or at other medical facilities such as hospitals and clinics. A copy of this type of form can be found at the end of this book. Please feel free to make copies for personal use.

The medical record is your life and health on paper. Once you get your records, it is important to review them for accuracy. If any information is inaccurate or any reports are missing, bring it to your doctor's attention. You might find some things your doctor did not tell you about or things you simply do not understand. If your doctor is unable to get the missing information, contact the source directly for copies of your reports.

Gather this information into a folder or notebook. Add a cover sheet with your name, address, phone number, email, and date of birth. On this page make a list of your medical conditions, all the medicines you take, your allergies (and any other reactions to medication), operations you've had, and a history of diseases that run in your family. You will be able to make copies to take to any doctor you go to. This also prevents the delay that occurs when records are sent from doctor to doctor, which can take from weeks to months to years.

CHAPTER 2

THE DOCTOR VISIT

As a patient, there are certain things you must know to be sure you are getting the proper medical care and the most professional treatment that all people deserve regardless of cost. In the medical world there is, however, a real cost. One goal of many health providers is to care for patients at a lower cost. Another goal is to provide the best care possible in a timely manner. This is called "cost-effective quality care." It can be done, but the important thing is to do it without compromising the quality of healthcare. This includes prevention, early detection, and proper treatment. These things must be done regularly and accurately. Much of the process must be managed by you, the patient. It is up to you to do what you can to be sure you are getting the best medical care and to have all the information to make the best medical choices for you.

Appointments

The doctor in charge of your overall care is called a primary care physician (PCP). Your first office visit with a new doctor is the most important one. This is when you get to know your doctor and supply information about your medical background. This visit may be for a specific problem or for a complete checkup (that is, a complete physical exam—CPE). For a specific problem, you might only get an examination of your complaints, symptoms (what is bothering you), and of other areas that the doctor knows to check depending on your symptoms. In this case, you are usually given a later appointment (typically in two to six weeks) for the CPE, but ideally you would have the CPE on your first visit. It is a good idea to make an appointment with your doctor while you are well. This will help you and your physician focus on your total healthcare more clearly and without distraction.

Schedules usually have 15-, 30-, and 60-minute time slots. The longer times are usually for patients who need a CPE. When you call for your first appointment, let the doctor's office know if that is what you want. That way you will not be put in a 15-minute slot, the time usually allowed for a routine visit. Doctors' schedules can be very frustrating for patients, doctors, and staff. This can lead to longer waits and shorter visits. Being on time is important for both patients and doctors.

Unless an emergency arises, the wait to see the doctor should be no longer than thirty minutes. If there is an emergency, waiting patients should be given the option of continuing to wait, rescheduling, or going elsewhere for treatment. If you really have to see the doctor, just be prepared to wait, and pray that the magazines are up-to-date. You can bring your own items to read, your laptop, a CD or tape player with earphones, or you can strike up conversation with other patients. Listening and talking with others in the waiting room is a great way to gather and share information. Also, take the time to observe. Take a look around the doctor's office and watch how things take place.

Some of the many reasons for a doctor's "tardiness" include overbooking patients, double booking (scheduling two patients at the same time), "pre-booking" (scheduling appointments before the doctor gets in), and emergencies. If you belong to a managed healthcare plan like an HMO (Health Maintenance Organization), the doctor usually has little, if any, say over the schedule because success is equated with seeing as many patients as possible. Also, the doctor may be an employee. The doctor who works for someone else cannot be solely blamed because the staff also works for someone else. Before managed care most doctors ran their offices and hired employees themselves. This means that the doctor was responsible for the whole office and the way it was managed. If your doctor is an employee and waiting is an issue, please let the doctor, office supervisor, and health plan know what has happened. The doctor will then be in a position to let the employer know there is a scheduling problem. This should help improve wait time and any related problems.

The History and Physical

The history and physical (H and P) form the cornerstone of good, quality medical care. The history is when the patient tells her or his medical story, and the doctor receives important information. Before the doctor gets started, a medical assistant or nurse will usually take your vital signs. These include temperature, weight, height, blood pressure, pulse, and respiration. Some doctors choose to have routine blood tests (which will be discussed later) done before they see you, whereas others choose to have it done afterward. This can be done in the exam room where the doctor will be seeing you, or the doctor may also have a special room set aside for taking vital signs and drawing blood. If blood tests are not done at the doctor's office, you might be sent to an outside laboratory or local hospital.

The Doctor Visit

Now you get to meet the doctor. The doctor will usually greet you by name and introduce herself or himself. Then, the doctor will want to know why you made your appointment. After you have answered, there will be questions from the doctor about your general health and wellness, as well as more information about your reason for the visit. For specific concerns you may be asked:

- How long has this been going on?
- What have you done for it?
- Have you had it before?
- Where does it bother you?
- How often does it occur?
- What makes it better or worse?
- Are there any other symptoms?

The doctor may then ask questions about how the other parts of the body are working, such as your eyes, ears, heart, breathing, and so on. This is called the "review of systems" (ROS). If there are any problems not related to your main problem, now is the time to let the doctor know.

This will be followed by your past medical history (PMH), which includes:

- Diseases you have (high blood pressure, sugar diabetes, arthritis, cancer, depression, etc.), or have had that are better or gone (including childhood diseases such as measles, mumps, and inherited disease)
- Operations and times you were in the hospital (including accidents)
- Medication, including prescription, over-the-counter (don't forget about vitamins), natural (garlic, aloe), and herbal
- Allergies and reactions to anything and what it did to you (for example: breaking out in a rash, swelling, itching, upset stomach, etc.)
- Smoking, alcohol, drug use (how much, how often)
- Shots (childhood, flu, last tetanus, etc.)
- Sexual (active, using protection, number of partners, diseases)—in females this will also

include menstrual period, pregnancy, last
mammogram, and Pap test

- Family history (conditions that run in family
such as cancer, high blood pressure, etc.)
- Social history—your job or jobs; family;
marital status; living arrangement (house,
apartment, alone, etc.); transportation (drive
self, public transport, walk); ambulation
(use walker, wheelchair); disability (deaf,
blind, amputee, etc.)
- Religion, ethnic customs, and traditions

If there is anything left out or that you feel the
doctor should know, now is the time to speak up.
It is sometimes hard to get someone's full
attention, so take advantage of it while you have
it. Some doctors' offices will have you fill out
forms asking the above questions or will ask you
the questions and fill out the form for you. This
is *not* a substitute for the doctor's personal
interview and questions.

The physical exam comes next. If you need a
CPE or an exam requiring part of your clothing to
be taken off, the doctor will now leave the room
for you to undress. Sometimes patients are fully
undressed and in the gown during the history
taking. This may save time (whose I'm not sure).

It is not comfortable or courteous. The gown or drape you will put on may be lying on the exam table, or the assistant may come in to help you get ready. If you need help with putting on the gown or getting on the exam table, this should be noticed. If not, ask for help. Getting on some of those exam tables is tricky, and putting on some of those gowns is trickier still.

Let the physical begin! First, I must let you in on a little secret. The doctor started your physical exam from the time you were greeted just by looking at you. Are you able to get up and shake hands? Are you able to sit back down? Is there a cane or walker lying beside you? Are you speaking clearly? Are you tearful? This and many other observations can tell the doctor a lot. So the physical has begun before the doctor puts a healing hand on you.

The head, eyes, ears, nose, and throat (HEENT) are usually inspected first. The doctor looks at the scalp for any hair loss or other abnormalities. Your head is palpated (touched and felt) to check for any lumps, swelling, or sore spots. The eyes are next. You will be asked to follow the doctor's finger with your eyes up, down, left, right. This tests your eye muscles. Pulling down the lower eyelid and pulling up on the upper eyelid allows for inspection of the white of the eye and the eyelids. The eye reflex is checked by shining a light on the colored part of the eye and is done with the lights dimmed (or light off and door cracked). The doctor uses the ophthalmoscope (an instrument) to look inside the eye. The blood vessels and nerve to the eye can be seen. Certain abnormal findings in the eye indicate diabetes, high blood pressure, and other maladies. For any findings that are abnormal with the eye, you will be sent ("referred" is the up-to-date term) to an ophthalmologist (eye specialist). Routine eye exams by the ophthalmologist may also detect some diseases that are known to progress toward blindness or other complications. Looking at and reading from an eye chart tests the vision.

Can you hear a whisper? How about a watch ticking? Faint noises close to the ears allow a doctor to check to see how well you can hear. Formal hearing tests (like audiometry) are done by an otolaryngology doctor, also known as the ENT (short for ear, nose, and throat) doctor. Hearing tests may also be done by hearing aid centers. The doctor uses the otoscope (the same instrument used for the eyes with an attachment made for looking in the ears) to look in the ear canal and at the eardrum. Using the same tool, each nostril and the mouth are inspected. A stick called a tongue blade is used to hold the tongue down when the doctor asks you to say "aaaaahhhhh." This is done so that the throat and the rest of the mouth can be checked. This procedure also tests the nerve for the gagging reflex (part of the nervous system exam). A gloved finger may be used to palpate (touch) the inside of the mouth. Any problems here will earn you a referral to the ENT doctor or dentist. Now may be a good time to ask any questions about the exam thus far. Please wait for the doctor to remove the gloved hand first.

The neck exam is next. At this time the thyroid gland is palpated. This is best done while the doctor stands behind the patient and places the right hand around the right side of the neck and the left hand on the left side of the neck. If any swelling or lumps are noted, further blood tests and a thyroid and/or neck scan may be ordered by the doctor. The lymph node glands can also be checked at this time. They are located in the front, back, and sides of the neck. They are also in the armpit and groin and are checked with those parts of the body. The lymph nodes should not normally be enlarged. More blood tests and X-rays may be ordered if they are enlarged.

Inspection, palpation, and percussion (lightly tapping) as well as listening to the chest give the doctor a chance to check the lungs. The doctor listens with a tool called a stethoscope, which makes the sounds louder. It is placed on the bare skin (beware of the doctor who tries to listen on top of your clothes) starting at the top of your upper back moving from the left to right, or right to left, from the top to the bottom of the chest while you take deep breaths. The same will be done on the chest. Then the stethoscope will be placed over the heart on the left and right sides of the breastbone. These areas are where the heart valve sounds are heard best. You may also be asked to do certain things like holding your breath or bearing down (as when having a bowel movement). This makes some murmurs easier to hear. Certain positions may also be better for hearing some heart sounds. Your doctor has been trained to listen for certain things. If any abnormal sounds are heard, more tests may be ordered. These may include an X-ray of the chest (CXR, for short) and heart tracing (electrocardiogram—EKG, for short). Usually these can be done in the office after completion of the exam. Depending on your complaints, symptoms, and the results of the CXR and EKG, you could require more tests that are not done in the primary care physician office. These tests will be discussed in the "Tests" and "Specialist" sections.

The breast exam is also done at this time. The doctor will let you know exactly what is to be done. For female patients, *it is recommended that a third person or chaperone be present when this exam is done.* After the gown is lowered to the waist, the doctor looks at the breasts with the patient sitting up on the exam table. The breasts should look the same size (sometimes one can normally be a tad larger or smaller than the other) and shape with the nipple positioned centrally. The breast is also checked to make sure there is no abnormal swelling, lumps, skin discoloration, or skin changes. Next you will be asked to put your hands on your hips and then raise your arms above your head much like doing your own breast inspection in front of the mirror. The doctor will again look and examine for any abnormal places. While you lie down on the exam table, the doctor will palpate each breast up and down vertically from right to left or vice versa. Palpation in a circle from out to in is another technique used. Breast tissue under the arm is also checked. The nipples are then squeezed gently to check for any discharge. Deeper palpation of the axilla (armpit) is then performed to check the lymph node glands. These steps are then repeated on the opposite breast. Any abnormalities may warrant a mammogram and/or sonogram (discussed further under tests) and possibly a surgeon's evaluation. Men should also receive a breast exam. This is a good time for the doctor to teach you to do your own self breast exam (SBE).

Now it's time to look, listen, tap, and feel the abdomen, the area many people refer to as the stomach. This is where the liver, spleen, kidneys, bowels, and female reproductive organs are located. With this lineup of important organs the doctor has a lot to check. This part of the exam is done in the supine (lying on your back) position. Looking at the abdomen for scars tells about any surgery you may have had. Listening with the stethoscope for overactive or underactive bowel sounds and/or bruits (sounds made by abnormal blood flow through arteries when there is blockage) is next. By tapping and feeling, a doctor is able to check for enlargement of the vital organs listed and to make sure that there are no abnormal internal masses or swelling. At this time the groin is also checked for any enlarged lymph nodes. If there are any abnormalities, further tests will be ordered by the doctor.

For females, the pelvic exam and rectal exam are next. The pelvic exam can also be done by a gynecologist, a doctor who specializes in female medicine. This depends on your preference and/ or if your primary care doctor chooses to refer you. It is an examination of the female external (outer) genitalia (parts) and internal (inside) reproductive sexual parts. The first female exam should be done at any age if there are any symptoms. Routinely, the first pelvic exam is done once the female is sexually active (having sex) or 18 years of age. *It is recommended that a third person or chaperone who is an authorized health professional should be in the room for this exam. Every health care setting should have chaperone policies in place for gynecology exams. This should always be presented as an option, if there is no policy or law. Furthermore, it should be offered to a patient for the full physical examination, especially if the physician is the opposite sex of the patient.* The assistant will help you get in position. Your legs will be placed in stirrups (foot holders) that are at the end of the table. You will then slide your hips down until the buttocks touch the edge of the table. Your legs will then be able to relax apart. (Some doctors have more comfortable exam chairs.) For those who might not be able to do this, there is the frog-leg position. The heels are brought together while the legs are bent: the heels are, thus, brought as close as possible to the buttocks, like frog legs. For persons not able to assume either of these positions, referral to a gynecologist is necessary. Please note also that you should *not* be put in this position until the doctor is ready to examine you. That's just good manners on the doctor's part. Once the exam begins, the doctor will instruct you when to lie down. You should also be informed when and where you will be touched during each part of the exam. The doctor will be wearing latex gloves to do this part of the exam. You may also request that a mirror be placed so that you can watch the exam.

There are five basic parts of the pelvic exam. The first part is the exam of the external genital area where the doctor inspects and palpates for any abnormalities. The second part of the exam is done using a tool called a speculum. This is for looking into the vagina and at the cervix. It resembles a fancy pair of tongs (or a pelican beak) and is either plastic or metal. Most doctors will and should warm the speculum with water before use. This allows for easier passage of the speculum. In the closed position the speculum is then placed gently in the vagina and opened to keep the vagina walls apart. When this is done, the doctor is able to see the cervix. The third part of the exam involves doing a Pap smear, which is a screening test for cancer of the cervix. A thin wooden stick about the size of a popsicle stick (called a spatula) and a stick with a tiny (about quarter-inch) brush on the end are used to do the test. When gently rubbed against the cervix, they are able to pick up cells. The cell samples are then placed on a glass side or in a test tube, which is then sent to the lab. The speculum is then removed.

Part four is the bimanual exam, which includes palpation of the internal female organs. One or two fingers that have been lubricated are placed in the vagina, while the other hand presses over the pelvic (lower abdomen) area. The uterus (womb) and ovaries (eggs) can be felt for any tenderness or masses. The last part of the exam is the rectovaginal exam. Using a clean lubricated glove, one finger is inserted into the vagina and a second finger into the rectum. This is an important part of the exam for two reasons: to check the rectum for bleeding and masses and to further palpate the female organs. *A complete pelvic exam includes a rectal exam.* The stool is checked for blood by placing a sample of stool from the gloved finger in the rectum onto a special card (commonly called guaiac or Hemoccult cards). If there is no stool for the specimen, your doctor will give you cards with instructions on how to collect samples at home. Once completed, the cards are returned to the doctor to be checked for blood. This is a very important test. Small amounts of blood in the stool cannot be seen with the naked eye but can be detected with this test.

The male genital exam is the equivalent of the female pelvic. The doctor inspects first. With gloved hands, the penis glans (tip) and shaft are checked. If the male is not circumcised, the foreskin (extra skin) should be pulled back. Then each scrotal sac is palpated to check the testicles for any abnormal lumps or bumps. This is a good time for the doctor to show you how to do your own monthly scrotal exam. Next the famous "cough" test is done in standing position. This is to check for hernias and is done with the insertion of the examining finger into the scrotal and inguinal (groin) area while the patient coughs. It is done on the right and left side. The rectal exam follows and is usually done with the doctor's lubricated gloved index finger inserted into the rectum. In addition to checking the stool for blood, the prostate gland (which makes male fluids) is also checked for size, tenderness, and masses. This is an important cancer screening test for men and should be done routinely after age 40.

Examination of the musculoskeletal system (arms, legs, back), nervous system (including mental health), and skin mark the end of the *complete* physical. The extremities (arms and legs) are checked for symmetry (the same on both sides) and deformity. Your ability to move was also checked as you got on and off the exam table, to see if you required assistance or were using an assistive device such as a wheelchair, walker, or cane. Following instructions and answering the doctor's questions during the exam allows for an indirect check of the nervous system. The skin can be inspected as each of the previous parts of the physical is done. Be sure to have the doctor show you how to do your own self skin exam.

The inspection of the extremities continues as the doctor looks for scars, skin color change, edema (swelling), and effusions (joint swelling). The joints of the arms and legs are then tested for range of motion (actual movement) actively (movements done by patient) and passively (extremities are moved by the doctor). They are also checked for any tenderness, swelling, and warmth or coolness. The strength, reflexes, and sensation (feeling) in the extremities are usually tested at this time or can be included in the neurologic (nervous system) exam. Strength is tested by resisting the doctor's strength. Pushing the hand against the doctor's hand, kicking the leg out, and gripping a finger with your hand are all relative tests of strength. The reflexes are checked with a reflex hammer at several places on the arm (front and back of the elbow, above the wrist) and leg (below front of knee, back of ankle on Achilles' tendon). Sensation can be checked using different items but is usually checked by light touch on the same parts of the arm or leg at the same time. A sterile pin touched lightly on the area to be checked can also be used. Different areas of the body are touched while the patient's eyes are closed and the doctor asks whether the touch feels the same on both sides or if a sharp or dull feeling is experienced with the pin. Position sense is checked by being able to tell if your finger or toe is being held up or down with eyes closed. Vibration sense is tested on a finger or toe joint with a tool called a tuning fork (a six-inch or so steel piece that vibrates when tapped lightly). Your job is to tell the doctor if it's vibrating and when it stops. Finally, the extremities are checked for the pulses (circulation) in the arm and leg and for any vein abnormalities.

The rest of the neurological exam involves checking the way you walk, talk, and answer a few questions designed to check the mental state (such as where you are, the date, ability to identify a simple object). The cranial nerves (nerves involving the face and neck area) can also be checked now, if they were not included in the head and neck exam.

During the back exam the doctor first looks at your posture. The shoulders and hips are checked for symmetry and deformities. The muscles of the neck, posterior thorax (chest), and lower back are palpated to check for any tenderness or spasm. Likewise, the bones of the spinal column are also checked. Movement of the neck and lower back is done actively and passively in all directions of movement.

Please be reminded that the way the physical exam is done may vary from doctor to doctor. This is unimportant as long as a *complete physical exam* is done. Please note that the above description of the CPE is quite generalized and does not include every specific detail. Book references for more detail include: *Bates Pocket Guide to Physical Examination and History Taking* by Barbara Bates, M.D., et al. (also available on CD-ROM and VHS tape), and *Bedside Diagnostic Examination* by Drs. Elmer and Richard DeGowan. Many medical school curricula use these references.

Once the physical exam is complete, the doctor and assistant will leave the room so you can get dressed. If an EKG (electrocardiogram—heart tracing) and X-ray are going to be done, you may be asked to get partially dressed (bottoms only) and keep the gown on. If blood has not been taken, that can be done at this time, too. Following these tests you will be able to get fully dressed.

The doctor will then sit down with you in the office or exam room and discuss your symptoms, the physical findings (normal vs. abnormal), diagnosis, and whether any further tests or treatments are needed. This is also the time for obtaining any prescriptions and to be told about any further tests or specialists whose expertise will be required. The doctor may also counsel you with information about your diagnosis and treatment, as well as any number of preventive healthcare topics. You may also be given handouts and booklets. Doctors may refer you to pertinent medical and patient education websites such as www.webmd.com. Email is becoming another way to talk with your doctor, in addition to phone calls, regular mail, and faxes.

Prescriptions for medication are usually given to the patient at the end of the visit. Prescriptions are written orders for medicine that the doctor has chosen for you. The patient should take these to the drugstore as soon as possible to stay well or to hasten recovery. Prescription medication must be dispensed by a licensed pharmacist. Some doctors fax or call the prescription in to your drugstore. Asking the doctor to do this for you will ensure you receive your medication promptly and will save you a trip to the drugstore. Some doctors are now using e-prescriptions over the computer to send in patient prescriptions. By giving your doctor the number for the druggist you use, you will be able to get a prescription filled in less time. You may also get prescriptions for medicine that can be bought over the counter—that is, without a pharmacist. Your pharmacist is the best person to help you with obtaining your medicine, discussing side effects and interactions, what the medicine is for, and so on. Be sure to discuss this with your doctor, too.

CHAPTER 3

PREVENTIVE CHECKUPS AND HEALTH MAINTENANCE

Staying healthy and disease-free is what prevention is about. The complete physical is the beginning of prevention. The breast exam checks for cancer, as do the Pap smear and rectal examination. Depending on your age and sex, there are guidelines for when to have certain tests. These guidelines are recommended by health organizations such as the U.S. Preventive Services Task Force, American College of Physicians, American Cancer Society, and American Heart Association. These guidelines are by no means laws, but they serve as useful suggestions for you and your doctor to use in your prevention and treatment program.

So how often should you have a complete physical? When is it time for your next tetanus shot? I have reviewed guidelines from the various health organizations mentioned above and compiled a summary of adult preventive care standards. These are also based on my own clinical experiences and on the number of lives saved by doing tests, regardless of whether the time frame of the guidelines was observed.

ADULT PREVENTIVE CARE STANDARDS

AGE:	18–25	26–40	41–60	60+
Physical Exam	1–3 years	1–3 years	1–2 years	yearly
Height/Weight	1–3 years	1–3 years	1–2 years	biannual
Blood Pressure	1–3 years	1–3 years	every year	biannual
Eyes and Ears	1–3 years	1–3 years	1–2 years	every year
Mouth	1–3 years	1–3 years	1–2 years	every year
Breast Exam	every year	every year	every year	every year
Pap Smear*	1–2 years	every year	every year	1–3 years
Prostate Exam	if needed	if needed	every year	every year
Scrotal Exam	every year	every year	every year	every year
Rectal Exam	if needed	if needed	every year	every year
Stool Blood Check	if needed	if needed	every year	every year

COMPLETE BLOOD PANEL

Lipid Panel	5 years	5 years	every year	every year
Liver Panel	5 years	5 years	every year	every year
Hepatitis Screen	5 years	5 years	every year	every year
Kidney	5 years	5 years	every year	every year
Blood Count (CBC)	5 years	5 years	every year	every year

*Some sources recommend that after two normal PAP smears, repeat every 1–3 years.

AGE:	18–25	26–40	41–60	60+
COMPLETE BLOOD PANEL, continued				
Thyroid	5 years	5 years	every year	every year
Urine	5 years	5 years	every year	every year
Electrolytes/ Minerals	5 years	5 years	every year	every year
Glucose	5 years	5 years	every year	every year
Prostate (PSA)	if needed	if needed	every year	every year
HIV	— — — test if any risk factors or exposure — — —			

IMMUNIZATIONS**

	18–25	26–40	41–60	60+
Tetanus- diphtheria	10 years	10 years	10 years	10 years
Pneumococcal	— as needed for persons at risk —			once after 65
Influenza (flu)	— as needed for persons at risk —			every year
Hepatitis	— — — — as needed for persons at risk — — — —			
Measles-Mumps-Rubella	— — if no antibodies, get 2nd dose — —			

TESTS / PROCEDURES

	18–25	26–40	41–60	60+
Mammogram	if needed	2–3 years	every year	every year
Chest X-ray (CXR)	baseline	if needed	if needed	if needed
Electrocardiogram (EKG)	— — baseline — —		every year	every year
Colonoscopy	if needed	if needed	3–5 years	1–3 years
Body Scan	baseline	1–3 years	1–3 years	1–3 years

DENTAL — — — — — — every year — — — — — —

MENTAL — — — — — — as needed — — — — — —

**For further details, refer to the "Recommended Adult Immunization Schedule" published by The Advisory Committee on Immunization Practices (ACIP) from the Centers for Disease Control and Prevention (CDC).

For any abnormalities, repeat screening and follow-up should be done sooner or more frequently depending on the individual person. For example, if your cholesterol is found to be increased when you are 18 years old or younger, you would want to have that checked at least every year instead of every five years. For people with a family history of breast cancer, yearly mammograms may start as early as the twenties. Persons with a history of chronic illness (diabetes, hypertension, cancer, etc.) should have a yearly physical regardless of age. Frequent routine visits during the year are also in order for those with any chronic illness. In addition to preventive health screening tests, preventive health counseling is also very important. In addition to the doctor's verbal counseling, ask for patient education references. Reading and knowing as much as you can about staying healthy also helps improve your quality of life and can make you feel better!

```
┌─────────────────────────────────────┐
│                                       │
│            CHAPTER 4                  │
│          ─────────────                │
│                                       │
│           MEDICAL                     │
│            TESTS                      │
│                                       │
└─────────────────────────────────────┘
```

CHAPTER 4

MEDICAL TESTS

Now that the doctor has talked with you and examined you, it is likely that more tests will be necessary. You may even need to be referred to a specialist, that is, a doctor that is an expert in a certain area of medicine. This chapter will guide you in explaining what the doctor has ordered and why.

Blood Tests

When the doctor orders blood tests (also called lab tests), she or he is checking for certain things. The most common tests are CBC (complete blood count), basic complete blood panel, and UA (urinalysis). The CBC checks the body's WBCs (white blood cells) and RBCs (red blood cells). In the lab the cells are examined for size, shape, and number. The WBCs may tell if you may have some type of infection or leukemia (cancer of the white cells). The RBCs carry oxygen to the rest of the body. This is done by hemoglobin, which is carried inside the RBCs. Some inherited diseases, such as sickle cell anemia and thallassemia, can be identified by abnormal RBC shape and size. Also included in the CBC is a platelet count. Platelets are cells that help your blood to clot, for instance to stop the bleeding after a flesh wound. The basic complete blood panel measures many different things. Included in these tests are:

- Na = sodium
- Cl = chloride
- K = potassium
- Mg = magnesium
- Glc = glucose (sugar)
- Ca = calcium (bone mineral)
- PO4 = phosphate (bone mineral)
- BUN = blood urea nitrogen (kidney)
- Cr = creatinine (kidney)
- SGOT = serum glutamic oxaloacetic transaminase (liver)
- SGPT = serum glutamic pyruvic transaminase (liver)
- GGT = gamma glutamyl transferase (liver)

- Alk phos = alkaline phosphatase (liver, bone primarily—also gallbadder)
- Fe = iron
- TIBC = total iron binding capacity
- transferrin = iron
- uric acid = checks gout
- chol = cholesterol (fat)
- LDL = low density lipoprotein ("bad" cholesterol)
- HDL = high density lipoprotein ("good" cholesterol)
- TG = triglycerides (fat)

Blood panels may differ from lab to lab. The above tests make up the basic chemistry panel. This should be part of a routine checkup. Some panels may include more tests than those listed above. The urinalysis (UA) may or may not be included, but it is important. Urine tests are able to check for infection, sugar, blood, protein, and many other things. Additional tests that may be ordered by the doctor for preventive screening will depend on your symptoms, diagnosis, family history, and age. Some of these tests are:

- PSA = prostate specific antigen (prostate cancer test)

- TSH = thyroid stimulating hormone (thyroid function)
- T4 = thyroid hormone (thyroid hormone level)
- B_{12} = vitamin B_{12}
- folate = B vitamin

Other tests than those listed may be checked depending on your history and physical exam. Be sure you are scheduled for a return visit to follow up on all tests. Some doctors' offices will also let you know by phone or mail, especially if there is an abnormal test that must be checked before your next appointment.

The Pap smear test and stool for occult blood (blood in stool that cannot be seen with the naked eye) should also be performed. The Pap smear, as mentioned earlier, is a test for females to check for cancer of the cervix. The stool test, also called Hemoccult test, checks for blood in the stool, which may indicate bleeding from the bowels secondary to cancer, ulcers, or other serious conditions. Details of both these tests were discussed in Chapter 2.

Other Tests

Your symptoms, the doctor's physical findings, and blood test results are what the doctor looks at when deciding the next tests that need to be done. This section will focus on the most common tests that your doctor may order. They may be used for screening, diagnosis of conditions, and for ongoing management of disease once it is present.

EKG

This test, also known as an electrocardiogram, gives information about your heart. It is usually done by the primary care doctor as part of a routine physical, especially if heart disease runs in your family. Typically, this test is done on anyone complaining of chest pain or discomfort. Small patches with adhesive on the back are placed on the chest, arms, and legs while the patient lies on her or his back. The electrode patches are attached to the wire cables running from the EKG machine. The heart's electrical activity is recorded on paper. By looking at this "heart tracing" graph, the doctor can tell if there are any abnormalities like irregular heartbeats (called arrythmias), damage to heart muscle from a heart attack, poor blood flow to the heart that causes chest pain (called angina), and heart enlargement. The doctor has been trained to know what changes or abnormalities need further testing, treatment, or hospitalization.

X-Ray

This test uses small amounts of radiation through an X-ray machine to make pictures. It can be done on almost any part of the body to check out a patient's symptom, and/or the doctor's findings during the physical exam. Many primary care doctors have X-ray equipment in the office. If not, the patient may be referred to a special office (diagnostic center) that performs X-rays or to a local hospital radiology department. X-rays are most commonly done on the chest, abdomen, back, joints, and extremities (arms and legs) and are done either with the patient lying down or standing up, depending on the part of the body being checked. After you have been positioned, the X-ray film cassette is placed in the machine next to the body part being X-rayed. The radiation from the machine will pass through the body part being X-rayed onto the film. The radiology technician (the person who operates the X-ray machine) will then move to a closed space in the same room and press the buttons to take the X-ray. During this test it is important that a protective lead shield apron be placed over the reproductive parts of the body.

Usually the technician will need to take more than one view, and so you will be asked to move a certain body part or turn a certain way. Different X-ray views give the radiologist (the doctor who reviews and interprets X-rays) a more complete view of the body part. Using the information from this test and the information from your history and physical, your doctor will be able to determine the proper diagnosis (what the problem is), treatment, and/or more tests, if needed.

There is some concern that the radiation from X-rays may be harmful. Studies have shown that small amounts of radiation are not linked with an increased risk of health problems. Over the years the amount of radiation used for X-rays has been decreased.

Ultrasound

This test is also referred to as a sonogram or sound wave test. The ultrasound uses sound waves to make images of body parts. This changes electrical energy to sound waves that go through the skin into your body. When the waves contact the body's organs, they reflect to the transducer, producing echoes. The echoes are then converted into still or moving images by a computer that makes a picture of your organs. The technician is able to see this on the monitoring screen and to make an X-ray or Polaroid-type picture. The ultrasound uses no radiation.

In this test the technician applies gel to the area to be tested. A transducer held by the technician is moved back and forth against that part of the body. This sends out the sound waves that go back into the computer. The sonogram is commonly used to look at your internal organs in the abdomen (such as the gallbladder, kidneys, liver, spleen, and pancreas), prostate, uterus, and ovaries. It is also used to look at blood vessels (arteries and veins), the thyroid gland, breasts, and the skull. In a pregnant patient, actual moving images of the fetus can be seen. As there is no radiation exposure, the sonogram is very valuable in following fetal development in pregnancy. It is also able to detect and diagnose other conditions related to pregnancy. Sonograms are also useful in checking the heart. These are called echocardiograms or Doppler echos.

Computerized Axial Tomography (CAT Scan, CT Scan)

The CT scan is another way to make images of body parts. The CT scanner uses X-ray beams that rotate around the body. These beams then go through a detector, and a computer analyzes and processes the data into an X-ray film. The CT machine has a table that is pulled in and out of the machine, which is a large hollow tube (like a doughnut) that can surround the body. During the test the patient lies down on the table. The scanner (inside the hollow tube) then rotates around the patient.

The CT scan is able to image many parts of the body. It detects more than a regular X-ray and produces two-dimensional views. This test is commonly used to pick up tumors, infections, enlarged organs, and many other abnormalities.

Magnetic Resonance Imaging (MRI)

The MRI scan is another diagnostic test that does not use X-rays. Instead, it uses magnetized energy. The images produced are extremely detailed pictures of the body part scanned. It is very much like looking at the pictures in an anatomy book or almost like looking at a person internally. The MRI machine is designed much like a CT scan machine, except a magnet is in the hollow tube instead of X-ray beams. The test is also done while the patient lies down on a table that moves in and out of the machine. The MRI scan takes about thirty minutes to an hour.

The MRI is not recommended for persons with metal or electronic implants (such as pacemakers, joint pins, prosthetics, artificial heart valves, metal fragments, shrapnel, IUDs, etc.), as those might interfere with the machine. Be sure your doctor and technician are made aware if you have any such implants. For the claustrophobic person, the closed space of the MRI machine may create some anxiety. Again, alert your doctor and technician. A mild sedative may be necessary prior to the test to help relax you, or you may be sent to a facility that has an open MRI. MRI scans are useful for scanning almost any body part for almost anything. Tumors, cysts, aneurysms, herniated back discs, and orthopedic conditions are among the many abnormalities that can be detected with this test.

Nuclear Scan

Nuclear scanning is also known as radioisotope scanning or radionuclide imaging. This test uses a radioactive substance called a tracer that is injected into the veins. The body is scanned with a special camera. This shows the uptake of the injected tracer by the body. Gallium scans use gallium citrate as the tracer; they are used for finding infections, inflammation, and cancer. Positive emission tomography (PET) scans are useful in diagnosing some cancers as well as heart and brain problems.

Mammogram

The mammogram is a plain X-ray picture of the breast. It requires a special machine that compresses each breast against X-ray film to take the picture. The X-ray passes through the breast tissue and shows how the breast looks inside. This test is excellent for detecting tumors and cysts. It may also show if the area is benign (no cancer) or malignant (cancer). The mammogram is able to pick up cancers that are too small to be felt or seen. It is a valuable cancer screening test.

Upper Gastrointestinal (UGI)/ Barium Enema (BE)

The UGI (upper intestine including esophagus, stomach, and small bowel) and BE (lower intestinal series) are X-ray tests of the bowels. Both tests require that barium (a substance that highlights the bowels during an X-ray) be taken. In the UGI the barium is swallowed. For the BE the barium is put into the rectum like an enema. Both of these tests require fasting (having nothing to eat or drink) after midnight the night before the test. For the BE one will also have to take a mild laxative and enema the day before the test. This is to empty and clean the bowel for better visualization. Most doctors provide written and verbal instructions on bowel preparation. For the UGI, the patient drinks a cup or two of barium or gastrogaffin. If a small bowel follow through (SBFT) is ordered with the UGI, the substance is taken at fifteen- to twenty-minute intervals with more X-rays administered after these ingestions. This test makes it possible to see most of the small intestine.

The barium is given as an enema (per rectum) for the lower GI series. The patient lies on the X-ray table and is securely strapped to the table (as with a car seat belt). The X-ray table is then tilted at different angles so that the barium spreads throughout the bowels. X-ray pictures are then taken at timed intervals as the barium flows through the system. This technique allows for the barium to provide contrast. As barium passes through the bowel, it is outlined in white so that the bowels and any abnormal areas will show up. These tests are very helpful in diagnosing most bowel conditions, including ulcers, tumors, cancer, inflammation, and bleeding.

For GI symptoms such as abdominal pain, weight loss, diarrhea, change in bowel habits, or blood in the stools, the UGI, SBFT, or BE is usually the first X-ray test ordered. Sometimes your doctor may recommend direct examination (endoscopy or colonoscopy) of the bowels as the first test in evaluation of GI complaints. If so, you will be referred to a GI specialist.

Intravenous Pyelogram (IVP)

The IVP is a test that looks at the renal (also called urinary) system, which includes the kidneys, ureters (tubes that connect the kidneys to the bladder), and bladder. This test requires contrast similar to barium but is given by needle injection through a vein (or IV, which means intravenous). X-rays are then taken at selected time intervals as the dye goes through the renal system. It is important that your doctor and technician know of your allergies, especially if you are allergic to iodine (found in different types of seafood), which is in the dye.

This test provides valuable information about kidney function and size. It shows renal abnormalities like stones, cysts, tumors, and blockages. If the patient is allergic to iodine, there are other tests that can be done to check the renal system. The other tests include sonogram, CT scan, and MRI scan, which can be helpful in evaluating any abnormal areas found on the IVP.

Endoscopy

Endoscopy is a procedure in which the doctor is able to look directly inside a part of the body through a very small lighted hollow tube. It is like a long, thin telescope with a light in it. The specific procedures usually take their names from the body part being examined. For instance, colonoscopy indicates an inside look at the colon (large bowel), and bronchoscopy is an examination of the bronchial tubes in the lungs. These procedures usually require mild to full sedation, which is given intravenously before endoscopy starts. The procedure may take anywhere from thirty minutes to an hour. Endoscopy tests are usually done on an outpatient basis at a diagnostic center or hospital. If there are no complications, the patient is able to go home the same day. Common types of endoscopy are as follows:

- arthroscopy—joints
- bronchoscopy—the trachea (windpipe) and bronchial tubes of the lungs
- colonoscopy—the colon (large bowel)
- cystoscopy—the bladder
- gastroscopy/upper endoscopy—the esophagus (swallowing tube) and stomach
- hysteroscopy—the uterus
- laryngoscopy—the larynx (voice box)
- laparoscopy—the abdomen

Endoscopy provides a direct view of the body system being examined and is also the best way to do a biopsy (that is, take a tissue sample of areas that look abnormal). A biopsy can detect cancer, tumors, and other diseases. Many operations that once required a large incision in the abdomen are now done with the laparoscope. It is inserted through the abdominal wall with a much smaller incision of an inch or less. Additional small incisions are made to insert surgical tools that may be needed for the surgery. Surgery done this way usually takes less time, and the patient goes home the same day as long as there are no complications. Recovery time is several days as opposed to several weeks after open surgery.

Body Scan

The electron beam tomography (EBT for short) body scan is a total scan of the body from the neck to buttocks area. This scan actually takes an anatomical picture of the body's internal organs. It takes about fifteen minutes or less depending on the type of scanner. This is an ideal screening test because it gives so much information in minimal time. The use of this test is very controversial. Ongoing studies are revealing that it is indeed a valuable screening tool. For instance, if there is a history of heart disease in your family, the heart scan would be able to detect and follow its progression or regression. It shows the heart vessels and is able to detect any narrowing or blockage (called calcium deposits, or plaque buildup from fat deposits in the heart vessels). The scan is very specific and is able to find abnormalities that might not show up on other scans. This has caused quite a bit of controversy in the medical community because it detects things that do not always need treatment. Some doctors feel it will lead to more unnecessary tests with more risks. The body scan is covered by some insurance plans and by Medicare for specific diagnoses or you can pay for it yourself. Average costs are from $700–$1,500.

This chapter has covered some of the most common tests you are likely to encounter as a patient. Along with your history, physical, and blood analysis, these tests provide the doctor with the information needed to make a correct diagnosis. Some of the tests are also used for maintenance and preventive purposes—that is, to keep you well. After the results have been reviewed by your doctor, she or he will be able to discuss them with you. If the tests done are not conclusive or your doctor is unable to make a diagnosis, you may be sent to a specialist.

CHAPTER 5

DOCTORS AND SPECIALISTS

For many people, the most familiar doctor is their personal or primary care physician (PCP). This is the doctor that coordinates all of your medical care routinely and continuously. Usually this doctor is a medical doctor (MD) who is a family practitioner, an internal medicine doctor (internist, for short), or a doctor of osteopathic medicine (DO). There may be times when your doctor or you feel an "expert" opinion is needed in a certain area. Then your doctor will refer you to a specialist. These doctors help the primary care physician with proper diagnosis and treatment. This section will focus on the most commonly used specialists.

Specialist Requirements

After completion of undergraduate and medical school in the United States (which usually takes from six to eight years), the physician enters an internship (first professional year) followed by a residency program (two years or more) at an accredited university program in the specialty chosen. The choice of specialty determines how long the doctor is in residency training. Family practitioners and general osteopathic doctors must complete three years of medical training in all areas of medicine. D.O.'s receive additional training in osteopathic manipulative medicine (OMT), which adds a holistic approach. Surgeons have three years of general surgery, including some general medicine. General internists train for three years. If a doctor chooses to specialize further, in a sub-specialty, there may be an additional two years or more of training.

Once training is complete, the doctor may take a test to become certified in the chosen specialty. This is an indication that the doctor has excelled in a particular field and is ready to provide the best, most up-to-date medical care. The doctor must possess a license to practice medicine for the state(s) in which she or he practices. This comes from the state licensing board, which also monitors physician conduct and competence. Doctors who do not follow the law are sanctioned by this board. The mission of the board of medicine is to protect the patient. Patients are able to contact the state boards to determine if doctors are licensed and if any disciplinary action has been taken against the physician for wrongdoing of any kind. In addition to providing information about physicians, the state boards handle patient complaints about doctors. This can lead to hearings where doctors are "tried" as in court and may lead to discipline and loss of license. The public information collected by state boards can be found on some state health agency websites.

Family Medicine

The family physician cares for the whole person and the whole family. Training in this specialty teaches one to care for all aspects of the patient no matter what age, sex, or illness. The Family Physician's Creed best describes this specialty, as follows:

> *I am a Family Physician, one of many across this country. This is what I believe: You, the patient, are my first professional responsibility, whether man, woman or child, ill or well, seeking care, healing or knowledge. You and your family deserve*

high quality, affordable health care including treatment, prevention and health promotion. I support access to health care for all. The specialty of family practice trains me to care for the whole person, physically and emotionally, throughout life, working with your medical history and family dynamics, coordinating your care with other physicians when necessary. This is my promise to you.

Because of their versatility, family doctors are often primary care doctors. They are able to diagnose and treat many different problems and refer to specialists when needed. They provide continuous routine medical and preventive healthcare . Family doctors may also perform minor surgical procedures in the office. These may include excision of small skin lesions such as warts, opening drainage of a small abscess, and even suturing (sewing up) minor lacerations like cuts. In addition, some also take additional training to perform procedures such as a colonoscopy.

Internist

An internist specializes in internal medicine for adults and adolescents. Like the family doctor, the internist provides routine medical and preventive care, functions as a primary care physician, and focuses on diagnosis and treatment of most general medical problems. The internist's three years of training include experience in non-surgical sub-specialties, such as allergy, cardiology, dermatology, endocrinology, gastroenterology, hematology, infectious disease, nephrology, neurology, oncology, pulmonary, and rheumatology. Other training includes emergency medicine, critical care medicine, hospital medicine, and geriatrics. After three years of training, the internist may decide to do additional training in a sub-specialty. Some of the most common specialists are described next.

Allergist (Immunologist)

An allergy doctor specializes in the diagnosis and treatment of allergies. Allergies occur when the body's immune (natural protection) system overreacts to something it's not used to being around, thus causing a reaction. Substances like pollen, certain kinds of food, mold, smoke, and medication may irritate a person's body: this is an allergy or allergic reaction. Symptoms may include an itchy rash, sneezing, a runny nose, and tears in the eyes. Shortness of breath, tightness in the chest, and wheezing indicate a more severe reaction, often requiring emergency treatment. When any of these symptoms are present, the primary care doctor may not be able to identify what is causing the reaction. This is when an allergy specialist is helpful. The allergist will recommend certain tests to find out the cause. Then a plan of treatment will be recommended, which may include oral medication, shots to decrease the allergy symptoms (called desensitization shots), and strategies for avoiding the things that cause the allergy.

Cardiologist

The doctor who specializes in the heart is called a cardiologist. Common reasons to see a cardiologist would include chest pain (angina), heart attacks, irregular heartbeats (arrhythmias), heart murmurs, abnormal EKG, hypertension, and pre-operative medical clearance. Tests performed by a cardiologist include EKGs, Doppler echocardiograms, and stress tests. Interventional cardiologists do "invasive" tests that involve entering the body through a blood vessel. These tests include cardiac catherization and angioplasty (opening blocked arteries). Each involves inserting a thin tube (catheter) into an artery to the heart. For the catherization, dye is injected through the catheter to outline the blood vessels.

This test will show any narrowing or blockage of the heart arteries. If the findings show obstructions, an angioplasty can be performed, which involves the insertion of a balloon catheter into the artery. Once inserted, the balloon is inflated to open the heart vessel. A stent (mesh tube) may be inserted and left in via the catheter to keep the artery open. This clears the artery, thereby relieving symptoms caused by angina or a heart attack.

Dermatologist

The specialist involved with treating the hair, skin, and nails is called a dermatologist. This type of doctor evaluates and treats skin rashes, growths, infections, hair loss, and nail abnormalities. Many diseases are associated with hair, skin, and nails. A dermatologist may be able to diagnose a specific disease based on a type of rash or a certain type of growth.

Emergency Medicine Specialist

The doctor who provides emergency care in a hospital emergency room (ER) or an emergency clinic is an emergency medicine specialist. The ER physician treats patients with acute illness who require immediate care. This includes conditions caused by trauma (car accident, fall, etc.) or sudden illness (high fever, chest pain, etc.) that may be life threatening.

Endocrinologist

Diagnosis and treatment of gland and hormone disorders is done by an endocrinology specialist. Specific organs included in the endocrine system are the thyroid gland (which regulates the body's metabolism and energy level), the parathyroid gland (which regulates calcium and Vitamin D), the adrenal gland (which regulates water and mineral balance, and makes some hormones), the ovaries (which regulate female hormones), the testes (which regulate male hormones), the pancreas (which secretes insulin to keep blood sugar in check), and the pituitary gland (which secretes precursor hormone releasers to other glands to make them work). The endocrinologist treats specific disorders associated with overproduction (hyper-) and underproduction (hypo-) of gland hormones.

Gastroenterologist

A gastroenterologist is a specialist trained to diagnose and treat conditions that affect the esophagus, stomach, small and large intestine, liver, gallbladder, and pancreas. Abdominal pain is one of the primary reasons this doctor is called upon. Abnormal abdominal tests of the gastrointestinal tract (GI) also require the expert opinion of the gastroenterologist, as endoscopy of the GI tract may be the next step in an evaluation. Endoscopy is also important in looking for causes of bleeding, such as inflammation, ulcers, tumor growths (polyps), and cancer.

Gynecologist/Obstetrician

Doctors specializing in women's medicine, including prenatal care and childbirth, are called obstetrician-gynecologists, gynecologist or obstetrician (depending on the need), or OB-GYN (pronounce each letter). These specialists train for four years in the specialty with some internal medicine included. They are clinical specialists who also perform surgery.

Hematologist/Oncologist

The hematologist specializes in disorders of the blood such as anemia (low blood), leukemia (cancer of blood cells), inherited blood diseases (such as sickle cell anemia), and lymphomas (cancer of the lymph node gland). An oncologist specializes in cancer diagnosis, treatment, and management. Because of the overlap with hematology, these particular specialties are usually considered together. If a blood disorder or cancer is suspected, this kind of doctor helps to make the final diagnosis and recommendations for treatment, which may include a bone marrow biopsy (a sample of tissue taken from an area inside the bone called the marrow, where blood cells are made) and chemotherapy (drug therapy for cancer).

Hospitalist

If you are admitted to the hospital, the hospitalist will care for you during your stay. This practice started in the 1980s. Prior to that time, the usual practice was for your personal physician to care for you in the hospital as well as the clinic. Some personal physicians still do this, whereas others use hospitalists. If you are admitted to the hospital, usually your primary care doctor is notified through your insurance plan. The PCP will discuss your case with the doctor who takes care of you in the hospital, and they will follow your progress jointly.

Infectious Disease Specialist

For infections that have not responded to treatment by your primary care, an infectious disease specialist is the expert for treatment. This doctor specializes in the diagnosis and treatment of infections caused by bacteria, viruses, and fungi, or that are of unknown origin. Common reasons for referral to this kind of specialist are life-threatening infections such as HIV and tuberculosis (TB) and others that are not responding in spite of treatment by your PCP.

Nephrologist

Nephrologists specialize in the diagnosis and treatment of kidney (renal) and urinary tract diseases. Any abnormalities in kidney blood tests, urine tests, and/or diagnostic kidney tests are referred to a nephrologist. These doctors are also trained to do kidney biopsies (tissue sampling) and to monitor patients on dialysis. Dialysis is a treatment for cleaning the blood through a special machine that removes toxins from the body as a result of kidney failure. The nephrologist also consults with the surgeon performing kidney transplants and related surgeries. If endoscopy of the renal system is necessary, the patient is also referred to a urologist.

Neurologist

Nervous system disorders, which include the brain, nerves, and spinal cord are managed by a neurologist. The patient history along with abnormal physical findings of the nervous system can provide clear indications for the necessity of referral to a neurologist. Symptoms and findings such as headache, weakness in arms or legs, "pins and needles" feelings (paresthesias) in arms or legs, and muscle twitches need to be investigated further. Neurologists specialize in brain disorders such as Alzheimer's disease, Parkinson's disease, seizure disorders, multiple sclerosis, brain tumors, and brain infections.

Ophthalmologist and Optometrist

Two types of doctors specialize in eye care: an ophthalmologist and an optometrist. Disorders of the eye and the correction of visual abnormalities are the focus of these doctors. This includes nearsightedness, farsightedness, and many other visual problems. Diseases such as high blood pressure and diabetes may cause eye disease that progresses toward blindness. Persons with systemic diseases that may cause visual problems see an ophthalmologist on a routine basis. Eye conditions such as glaucoma, macular degeneration, and cataracts also warrant close follow-up by the eye specialists. The doctor who studies ophthalmology is also trained to do eye surgery. Ophthalmologists may also choose to sub-specialize in specific eye diseases.

Optometrists (ODs) attend a college of optometry instead of medical school. They do not perform eye surgery, but they do examine, diagnose, and treat many of the same eye problems as the ophthalmologist. Optometrists are more involved in eye exams for glasses and/or other corrective aids. Opticians are healthcare professionals who are trained at technical school to help eye doctors. They dispense and fit corrective visual wear such as glasses and contact lens.

Pain Management Specialist

If you are having pain, there is a specialty that treats all types of pain. Pain management specialists are usually anesthesia doctors (who put you to sleep for surgery) with special training in pain management. Other doctors like family practitioners and internists are also becoming involved in this specialty. Chronic pain (defined as pain that lasts longer than three months) is managed by specialists on an outpatient basis for many conditions, especially those patients who have not responded to basic pain care. Treatments include the use of pain medication, needle injections in painful areas, and referrals for other types of therapy that may help, such as physical therapy, massage, acupuncture, etc.

Pathologist

In the specialty of pathology the doctor does not provide any clinical care or "hands on" patient care. The pathologist examines tissue specimens (biopsies) from the body. For example, when a doctor takes a tissue sample from an area that looks abnormal or suspicious, the sample is taken to the pathology lab. The pathologist takes a closer look with a microscope.

The pathology specialist also oversees the laboratory personnel who handle blood and other bodily fluids that require testing. Forensic pathologists perform autopsies.

Pediatrician

Although the primary focus of this book is on adult medicine, the pediatric specialty deserves mention, for adults with children (or grandchildren) will have contact with them too. The pediatrician specializes in newborn, infant, child, and adolescent medicine. There are sub-specialties of pediatrics, as in adult medicine, such as the pediatric nephrologist, neurosurgeon, anesthesiologist, psychiatrist, etc.

Podiatrist

Foot disorders are diagnosed and treated by podiatrists. A doctor of podiatric medicine (DPM) also performs surgery related to the foot and ankle. Podiatrists treat problems such as ingrown toenails, bunions, corns, and physical deformities of the foot and ankle. They also perform routine foot checks (including toenail cutting) for those at risk of developing foot ulcers, such as diabetics and those with poor circulation.

Psychiatrist

The psychiatrist is the specialist who diagnoses and treats mental well-being and mental disorders such as anxiety, depression, phobias, etc. The psychiatry specialist also deals with behavioral problems. Counseling and psychotherapy are among the services a psychiatrist provides.

Pulmonologist

The pulmonologist specializes in pulmonary medicine, which treats the lungs and chest. Asthma, chronic obstructive pulmonary disease (COPD, for short—a disease caused by smoking), lung cancer, and pneumonia are common conditions this doctor diagnoses and treats. Abnormal chest X-rays and chest scans are also referred to this specialist. Diagnosis may require a bronchoscopy, which may be done by the pulmonologist.

Radiologist

Interpretation of X-rays and other diagnostic studies (such as MRI, CT, sonogram, mammogram, etc.) are done by the radiologist. Some diagnostic X-ray tests require a doctor who specializes in radiology to perform the test as well as read the result. They are called interventional radiologists and perform procedures such as biopsies (taking tissue samples) and angiograms (dye studies of vessels).

Radiation Oncologist

A radiation oncologist is a doctor who specializes in the treatment of cancer using radiation. This doctor is specially trained to determine the area where the radiation goes, the type of radiation needed, and the dose for each type of cancer. The radiation oncologist works very closely with the oncologist and the primary care physician in the treatment of cancer.

Rheumatologist

A rheumatologist specializes in the diagnosis and treatment of conditions that affect the joints, muscles, and connective tissue (tissue that binds and supports parts of the body together, that is "connects"). Ailments the rheumatologist treats include arthritis, fibromyalgia, lupus, and any symptoms suggestive of rheumatism.

Surgeon

Training for a surgery specialty begins after medical school in a general surgery residency program. For the surgeon who wishes to sub-specialize, the training takes a few more years. General surgeons operate on "general" cases like appendicitis, gallstones, and hernias. Some of the more common surgery sub-specialties are listed and described below. For each body part and system there is a surgeon specialist. Some of these are:

- Cardiac/Cardiothoracic—heart, chest, lungs (thorax), and related structures
- Colorectal—large intestine, rectum, anus
- Hand—hand disorders and injuries
- Laparoscopic—abdominal surgery through a scope
- Neurosurgeon—nervous system, brain, nerves, spine
- Ophthalmic—eyes
- Oral—mouth, teeth, jawbone
- Orthopedic—bones, joints, spine
- Otolaryngology—ear, nose, throat, mouth
- Plastic/Reconstructive—cosmetic and replacement or reduction
- Vascular—blood vessels such as the aorta and other major vessels

Some of the sub-specialties may overlap in the type of surgery performed, especially with general surgery. For instance, a back problem like a slipped disc can be properly handled by an orthopedist or neurosurgeon. Some specialties have a medical and surgical training such as ophthalmology.

Urologist

The urologist specializes in surgery of the urinary tract—the kidneys, ureters (tube-like organs that connect kidneys to the bladder), and bladder. Prostate checkups and the treatment of prostate disorders are also part of this specialty.

Anesthesiology

When it's time to have an operation, the anesthesiologist is the doctor that puts patients to sleep or provides local anesthesia. The anesthesiologist follows the patient's condition during surgery by monitoring the blood pressure, respirations (breathing), heart rate, etc. Along with the surgeon the anesthesiologist also helps manage pain after surgery (post-operative pain). Some hospitals and outpatient surgical facilities use certified registered nurse anesthetists (CRNAs). CRNAs take care of patients in the same manner as anesthesiologists and give about 65% of anesthetics per year to patients in the United States. They are the only anesthesia providers in more than two-thirds of the nation's rural hospitals. Nurses must attend an accredited nurse anesthesia program and pass a national certification exam to become CRNAs.

Dentist

Dentists are doctors that care for the teeth and gums. Dental care includes routine checkups for prevention of tooth and gum disease, which they also treat. Some dental sub-specialties include orthodontics for braces, oral surgeons for operations, and cosmetic dentistry for improving teeth appearance.

Complementary Medical Specialists

The National Center for Complementary and Alternative Medicine (NCCAM) (an organization under the government's National Institutes of Health—NIH) defines complementary and alternative medicine (CAM) as "a group of diverse medical and healthcare systems, practices, and products that are not presently considered part of conventional medicine." Conventional medicine, also referred to as Western or traditional medicine, deals more with the treatment of disease and symptoms and the part or parts of the body involved. CAM focuses on treating the whole person (body, mind, and spirit) and preventing disease. Integrative medicine (IM) is a combination of conventional medicine and CAM.

CAM specialists include naturopathic doctors (ND), chiropractors, and osteopathic doctors (osteopathic medicine is also considered conventional). Naturopathic treatment uses CAM therapies to focus on maintaining and restoring health. Chiropractors focus on the body, especially the spine, primarily through manipulative techniques of the spine to maintain stable health. Osteopathic doctors feel that the body works together such that symptoms and disease in one part of the body affect the whole body function. They focus on the musculoskeletal system and use techniques on the whole body for healing. Traditional Chinese medicine (TCM) and Ayurveda are alternative treatments derived from Eastern medicine (China, India). Other CAM therapies include aromatherapy, massage, yoga, herbs, electromagnetic fields, acupuncture, homeopathy, and diet supplements. These can be combined with each other and with conventional medicine. Persons that specialize in these areas are required to do professional training and to obtain a license to practice.

According to an NCCAM survey in 2000 more than two-thirds of Americans use CAM. Prayer is the top CAM therapy, followed by natural products, meditation, and special diets. Many turn to CAM when they feel conventional treatments aren't or don't work or have too many side effects. Some patients prefer CAM treatment to stay healthy and feel they are more natural and safer. This deserves a word of caution, as only a few CAM treatments have been studied enough to prove that they work and are safe for use. Be sure to discuss any complementary or alternative treatments you use or plan to use with your doctors and other medical providers.

Physician Extenders

Physician extenders are health providers who help doctors. The primary ones are physician assistants (PA) and nurse practitioners (NP). These healthcare professionals do much of the same work as doctors but must work under a doctor's supervision. They are rapidly appearing on the forefront of primary care and specialty medicine. A physician extender may be the first person you see on an office visit to the doctor or prior to a procedure. After a patient is seen, the PA or NP presents the patient history and physical to the doctor and continues patient care with the doctor's supervision.

Some of the other medical providers you will encounter include nurses, nurse assistants, medical assistants, medical technologists, and medical therapists. All must be trained and licensed in their specialty. They help doctors in giving patient care in the office and hospital and as independent service providers (such as physical therapists, respiratory therapists, etc.), Many provide home care services and checkups. Like doctors, these professionals also work as administrators, consultants, and in other jobs that involve roles not associated with direct patient care.

CHAPTER 6

HEALTH INSURANCE AND QUALITY

Managed healthcare is the primary way health insurance is provided today. The basis of managed healthcare systems is to encourage prevention as well as provide treatment in a quality, cost-effective manner. Although studies have shown that managed healthcare lowers costs, these costs are still very high and steadily rising. As a result, doctors may be inclined to order fewer tests and patient referrals to keep costs down. Most of these health plans require the patient to have a primary care doctor, who becomes the provider and coordinator of the selected patient services. Costs may be contained, but quality may not be acceptable. In view of these ever-changing times of healthcare and its reform, a patient must be informed about the basics of managed healthcare.

Health Plans

Managed care plans include: health maintenance organizations (HMO), preferred provider organizations (PPO), and point-of-service (POS) plans. HMO health insurance is based on the capitation concept, a fixed payment per patient per month. This capitation fee, or insurance premium, may be paid by an employer, individual, physician group, or the government (as in Medicare and Medicaid). Doctors, hospitals, specialists, and other medical services are chosen by the HMO clinic owners. This means the patient is limited to receiving care from doctors whom the HMO has selected. The patient usually chooses or is assigned to a primary care physician (PCP) on the HMO selected list of providers. HMO clinics are like franchises, that is, individual clinics may be run by physicians and/or non-physicians who pay to be a partner with the HMO company. The HMO also contracts with private doctors or private group practices to provide services. This is called an independent practice association (IPA). It allows private doctors to have provider contracts with several HMO plans while also using indemnity coverage.

Medicare and Medicaid HMOs receive money from the government. The premium is derived from actuarial charts based on age, sex, and residential area. With these monies, contracts are made with HMOs to provide medical care to assigned patients. Each HMO franchise has its own contracted providers for necessary medical services. These are called provider networks, which consist of specialists, hospitals, diagnostic centers, pharmacies, and other medically necessary service providers. Often confusing to people is the fact that different HMO franchise clinics share the same franchise company name; however, these clinics are run by different people with different networks. Usually services are not interchangeable. This means that a patient is not able to go from HMO A's Clinic 1 to HMO A's Clinic 2 for service, unless they are owned by the same people. Patients are allowed to change to another HMO clinic if not satisfied with services from their present clinic. This usually has to be done by a certain time of month or year to be eligible for transfer by the first of the next month. This process is called disenrolling from the plan. There is a formal process by which this is done, and it may vary slightly from one HMO to another.

HMOs provide comprehensive services, including routine checkups, physicals, immunizations, hospitalizations, and preventive medical care. The services covered and not covered are outlined in the patient membership handbook, which should be provided to patients once enrolled. Some Medicare HMOs provide dental and eye care "free of charge"—that is actually included in the fixed monthly capitation rate. Some commercial plans also do this, but as medical costs rise, this practice is becoming less common. Insurance providers are now requiring a partial payment by the patient for almost all services. Coverage for some services, such as prescriptions, optometry, dental care, and office visits, may require a co-payment to be rendered at the time of service. This is usually $5 and up. It depends on the type of coverage provided by the insurance plan. Emergency room visits may also require co-payments.

Hospitalizations are usually covered 100% by HMOs, but they may require partial payment and a deductible. The deductible is the amount the patient is responsible for paying before the insurance starts paying. If the hospital stay is longer than necessary for the medical condition being treated, the patient may be responsible for payment. For example, the time an insurance plan allows for a heart attack may be five days in the hospital. The physician may feel extra days are needed, especially if complications arise or if the patient is not stable for discharge. To have this covered by insurance, the doctor may have to show that hospitalization is still necessary.

PPO (Preferred Provider Organization) insurance plans offer services very similar to those of an HMO. A PPO, however, offers more choices. The patient may use doctors, hospitals, and other medical services not on the PPO "preferred provider" list. The patient may have to pay extra if "preferred providers" that the PPO has selected are not utilized. In addition, the insurance premium may be higher than through an HMO, with a higher deductible amount.

POS (Point of Service) plans are another type of managed care where the patient can get services from providers that may or may not be from the plan's network of providers. If used as an HMO, the cost of a POS plan is minimal. If used as a traditional indemnity insurance, one is able to see the providers of choice but must also pay. PSO (Provider-Sponsored Organization) health plans are usually owned and operated by doctors and hospitals.

Indemnity health plans provide traditional, private fee-for-service insurance. They were the model of health insurance before managed healthcare began about twenty-five years ago. With this type of health plan, the patient chooses the doctor and other medical services and pays coinsurance, that is, a percentage of the fee (usually 20%). The insurance company pays the remainder and largest portion (usually 80%). If the amount billed is more than the usual charge paid by the insurance company, the patient must pay that difference too. Indemnity health insurance coverage involves payment of a monthly premium and may include deductibles before payment begins. Unlike in MCOs, the medical care is more focused on active, chronic health problems with less emphasis on wellness and prevention. You may get to use the doctors and hospitals you desire, but you may also pay more.

Medicare and Medicaid are government funded medical programs that provide health insurance to people over 65, those with end-stage kidney disease, and some disabled persons. Medicare is funded by the federal government.

Medicaid receives funds from the federal and state governments, and each state runs its own Medicaid program. Medicaid primarily provides coverage to those with low incomes. Some nursing home coverage is provided for the low-income elderly through Medicaid, also. There are HMOs for Medicare and Medicaid that provide medical care and services. Most states offer traditional Medicaid and Medicaid HMOs.

Personal health savings accounts (HSA) were introduced by the federal government in 2003 as part of the Medicare reform law. One must have a high deductible health plan (HDHP) to get an HSA. HDHPs have a higher deductible than traditional health plans. Benefits are paid after the annual deductible is met (except for preventive care). The health plan decides if you qualify for an HSA. Health reimbursement arrangements (HRA) are available for those who do not qualify for an HSA. This account is funded by the employer. It may also be obtained if you have Medicare or if you are covered by a plan that is not an HDHP. HRA credits cannot be carried over to the next year, nor do they earn interest like an HSA.

These are the basic types of healthcare coverage available today. For those without insurance coverage, payment for medical care is out of pocket. Some doctors and medical providers allow discounts and payment plans if you let them know you are uninsured and paying directly with cash, check, or credit card. If you are insured or uninsured, it is a good idea to include medical expenses in your monthly budget, along with other necessities such as food, rent, etc. Just because you do not have medical insurance does not mean you have to forgo medical attention.

Quality of Medical Care

Quality medical care can be described as the best medical care. The goal is to keep a person well and healthy and to manage acute and chronic illnesses to help a person maintain optimum health. According to a 1996 national survey, "Americans As Health Care Consumers: The Role of Quality Information," the major concern in choosing a health plan was quality of care (42% of 2,006 adults). This is more important than low cost, choice of doctors, and range of benefits. Employers provide some information on the quality of health plans. Most people choose health providers and health plans based on recommendations from doctors, family, and friends.

There are independent organizations such as the National Committee for Quality Assurance (NCQA) and the Agency for Healthcare Research and Quality (AHRQ) that monitor and provide information about the quality of healthcare. They develop and report their findings based on research. The AHRQ (www.ahrq.gov) is a government agency that supplies research and guidelines for use by health providers and patients to help determine what care is available and which should be preferred. The NCQA (www.ncqa.org) assesses, monitors, and reports on quality of care. It is a private, nonprofit organization whose diversified board of directors includes employers, health plans, and most importantly, patients, the consumers of managed healthcare. The Joint Commission on Accreditation of Healthcare Organizations (JCAHO) evaluates hospitals, clinics, nursing homes, home health agencies, and laboratories. For community, home health, and hospice programs there is the Community Health Accreditation Program (CHAP). Outpatient healthcare settings like student health services, diagnostic radiology centers, and ambulatory surgical centers are evaluated by the Accreditation Association for Ambulatory Health Care (AAAHC). In addition, most managed healthcare plans have their own internal quality assurance plans.

Once a plan has been reviewed and evaluated by NCQA or other review agencies, the plan is assigned a "grade." If the plan meets the required standards, it is then given accreditation. This means that the plan met the required guidelines for providing high-quality medical care. The NCQA uses this information to develop a report card on each plan it reviews. The NCQA measures quality using its own Health Plan Employer Data and Information Set (HEDIS) for performance measurement. This data is used for the report card. The report card includes data on the plan's actual medical services, such as doctor availability, specialist referrals, preventive care, and emergency and hospital coverage. It also reviews charts focusing on the physician's medical competence and performance. The physician's licensing, certification, and other credentials are also checked. The physical setting of the office is evaluated to be sure that all quality standards are met.

In evaluating healthcare quality NCQA accreditation and HEDIS provide a comprehensive, standardized, and uniform method that is used for the HMOs it reviews.

About 75% of the nation's HMOs are accredited by NCQA or are in the process of becoming accredited. The following areas are the primary focus of the health plan review, weighted according to the percentages indicated:

- Access and service (patient satisfaction and easy, timely access to providers and treatments), 40%
- Qualified providers (trained, licensed, credentialed), 20%
- Staying healthy (wellness and prevention), 15%
- Living with illness (proper diagnosis and treatment of acute and chronic medical problems), 15%
- Getting better (quality of care), 10%

Meeting the accreditation standards in each area accounts for 75% of the grade. The HEDIS (Health Plan Employer Data and Information Set) results make up the remaining 25%. Overall, HEDIS results look primarily at quality in the clinic and patient satisfaction. The results from each plan review are then compared to certain target goals for each category reviewed, and the plan is graded. These grades are compiled and compared to other health plan report cards. The collected information is then reported in a comprehensible format for patient use in selecting a quality health plan.

Information like this is becoming more readily available. It will become, increasingly, one of the ways patients look for and find quality health plans. The Accreditation Status List (ASL) is available to anyone by calling (1-888-275-7585), by writing , or by going to the NCQA website, which provides a list of the accreditation status of participating health plans. Accreditation Summary Reports (ASR) are also available and contain more detailed information than the ASL.

Individual private doctors and group practices that use these managed healthcare plans are usually under contract with the health plan to allow for periodic quality assurance checkups and monitoring. Health insurance that is not part of a managed healthcare plan and private fee-for-service healthcare are also being included in assessments of quality. Uniformity of quality assessment and reporting among all healthcare providers is a major issue being addressed by the government and other independent agencies that specialize in quality measurement. Soon all providers of all types of health services will have routine quality assessment and reviews, and even more information will be available for the patient to review.

Even with the researched, scientific-quality databases provided by independent organizations, patients usually select a health plan and providers recommended by family or friends rather than one that rates much higher based on a formal quality assessment and review. This trend is also reflected in the choice of doctors. Patients are more concerned about the way a doctor communicates with and cares about them than about whether the doctor has been given a high rating by a quality assurance organization. If the doctor has board certification in her or his specialty, this is also given a higher ranking by patients than quality accreditation from an independent organization.

Many people are beginning to see that quality is important, since one of the goals of managed care is to contain costs, sometimes at the patient's expense. In order to see that this does not become an issue, quality monitoring, assessment, and reporting are vital to the healthcare system. Making it available to the patient is also important. Information is a powerful tool. It allows patients to learn and to make decisions that are best for them. Looking for quality healthcare in today's healthcare maze can be a challenging experience. Reading information from the medical provider is a good place to start. Many managed health plans provide patient manuals and patient representatives that are available to talk with you in person or by phone. For more detailed information you can contact your state's insurance commission. Health insurance plans are regulated by state insurance commissions.

The AHRQ is a federal government agency under the Department of Health and Human Services (DHHS). It does research on the quality and costs of healthcare. Some of the specific healthcare areas it covers are patient safety, quality improvement, clinical outcomes, assessment of medical practices, preventive and primary care services, and funding for medical research. AHRQ states:

> *Health services research examines how people get access to health care, how much health care costs, and what happens to patients as a result of this care. The main goals of health services research are to identify the most effective ways to organize, finance, and deliver high quality care; reduce medical errors; and improve patient safety.*

The AHRQ has maintained a database of medical care guidelines based on medical research. The research is "translated" into practices and policies that have been proven to provide the best care, diagnosis, treatment, and follow-up for specific conditions. The guidelines are available free of charge at The National Guideline Clearing House (www.guidelines.gov).

More information on choosing the right health plan for your medical needs can be found in the following patient information brochures available on the Internet or by contacting the agency via phone or mail:

- "Choosing and Using a Health Plan" and "Checkup on Health Insurances" from AHRQ
- "Choosing Quality: Finding the Health Plan That's Right for You" from NCQA
- "Which Plan Is Right for Me?" from NCQA
- The www.healthchoices.org website by NCQA
- "It's Your Health—How to Get the Most Out of Your HMO" from Consumer Action, www.consumer-action.org, a consumer advocacy group

CONCLUSION

This book provides basic information to assist anyone with obtaining quality medical care. The topics covered provide the foundation for building solid health maintenance and ongoing medical care. The history and physical exam along with the routine tests we have considered are the first steps to establishing your health record. Keeping track of it yourself is important for self-motivation to stay healthy, practice prevention, and obtain early diagnosis and treatment. All of these things will help you maintain an excellent quality of life. The information provided here about tests, specialists, and the managed healthcare system will help guide you along the path to getting the proper care for any health problems that might arise.

With this handbook you are now ready to take action and more responsibility for your most important asset—YOU! You will be a more effective and active participant in your entire health plan by making informed choices and the best choices for your health. Start your medical diary now with your medical history. The blank pages at the back of this book are intended for that purpose. You can continue them in a notebook or on the computer. Begin managing your healthcare by using this book as a guide. Remember that prevention is better than a cure. Stay healthy!

MY HEALTH NOTES

_____

_____

_____

_____

_____

_____

_____

_____

_____

_____

_____

_____

_____

_____

_____

_____

_____

_____

_____

_____

_____

MY HEALTH NOTES

MY HEALTH NOTES

MY HEALTH
N O T E S

AUTHORIZATION FOR
RELEASE OF INFORMATION

AUTORIZACION PARA PROPORCIONAR INFORMACION

I HEREBY GIVE MY PERMISSION TO/Yo por este medio doy mi permiso a:

_____

_____

TO RELEASE A COPY OF (LIST SPECIFIC INFORMATION/DOCUMENTS)/
A que proporcione una copia de (liste informacion/documentos especificos):

_____

_____

_____

TO/A: _____
(AGENCY, MENTAL HEALTH PROFESSIONAL, ATTORNEY / Agencia, Profesional de Salud Mental, Abogado)

ADDRESS: _____

_____

_____

I HEREBY RELEASE THE FACILITY FROM ANY LIABILITY WHICH MAY ARISE AS A RESULT OF THE USE OF THE INFORMATION CONTAINED IN THE RECORDS RELEASED./Yo por este medio relevo a esta empresa de cualquier responsabilidad que pueda surgir como resultado del uso de le informacion contenida en los documentos remitidos.

NAME OF PATIENT/Nombre de paciente: _____

BIRTH DATE/Pecha de nacimiento:_____

SIGNATURE OF PATIENT/Firma del paciente: _____

DATE/Firma del testigo:_____

SIGNATURE OF GUARDIAN/Firma del custodio: _____

DATE/Firma del testigo:_____

(IF NEEDED/Si es necesario)

SIGNATURE OF WITNESS: _____

DATE/Firma del testigo_____   (more...over)

TO RECEIVING AGENCY: PROHIBITION OF REDISCLOSURE

A LA AGENCIA QUE RECIBA LA INFORMACION: PROHIBICION DE REVELAR

THIS INFORMATION HAS BEEN DISCLOSED TO YOU FROM RECORDS WHOSE CONFIDENTIALITY IS PROTECTED. ANY FURTHER REDISCLOSURE IS STRICTLY PROHIBITED UNLESS THE PATIENT PROVIDES SPECIFIC WRITTEN CONSENT FOR THE SUBSEQUENT DISCLOSURE OF THIS INFORMATION.

Esta informacion ha sido proporcionada a usted de documentos cuya confidencialidad es protegida. Cualquier declaracion adicional es estrictamente prohibida a menos que el paciente de su consentimiento especificamente por escrito permitiendolo.

Give the Gift of

PATIENT HANDBOOK
TO MEDICAL CARE
Your Personal Health Guide

to Your Friends and Colleagues

CHECK YOUR LEADING BOOKSTORE OR ORDER HERE

❑ **YES**, I want _____ copies of *Patient Handbook to Medical Care* at $16.95 each, plus $4.95 shipping per book (Florida residents please add $1.19 sales tax per book). Canadian orders must be accompanied by a postal money order in U.S. funds. Allow 15 days for delivery.

My check or money order for $_____ is enclosed.

Please charge my: ❑ Visa ❑ MasterCard
❑ Discover ❑ American Express

Name _____

Organization _____

Address _____

City/State/Zip _____

Phone_____ Email _____

Card # _____

Exp. Date_____ Signature _____

Please make your check payable and return to:
Bend of the River Books
P.O. Box 330645 • Miami, FL 33233-0645

Call or fax your credit card order to: 1-866-362-0411
www.mypatienthandbook.com